When You Can't Pour From an Empty Glass

CBT Skills for Exhausted Caregivers

Dr. Patricia A. Farrell, Ph.D.

Contents

Cover photo: Rak Ankong@unsplash.com

ISBN: 979-8-9986832-4-4

Books by Patricia A. Farrell, Ph.D.

How to Be Your Own Therapist

It's Not All in Your Head: Anxiety, Depression, Mood Swings and Multiple Sclerosis

Unfiltered: Beneath the noise of our thoughts lies the true narrative of our minds

Unfiltered Again: A behind-the-scenes look at healthcare, medicine and mental health

A Social Security Disability Psychological Claims Handbook: A simple guide to understanding your SSD claim for psychological impairments and unraveling the maze of decision-making

A Social Security Disability Psychological Claims Guidebook for Children's Benefits

The Disability Accessible US Parks in All 50 States: A Comprehensive Guide

Birding in the US NOW!: A birding guide for individuals with disabilities

Chapter One

Introduction: Welcome to a Journey of Care and Self-Discovery

Welcome. If you've picked up this book, it's likely because you find yourself in the demanding, often overwhelming role of a caregiver, and you are reaching out for help. Perhaps you care for an aging parent, a spouse facing chronic illness, a child with special needs, or someone else dear to you who requires daily support. You may not have expected or prepared for this situation. But it's here now, and you face an overly demanding role. Even if you didn't want to do this, you will because you have a connection that is very strong—it's love.

Love moves us in many directions, and it will guide you in the months and years to come.

First, I want you to know: **you are not alone**. The caregiving community is vast and growing, and you are part of a vital, compassionate network of people who give selflessly—often at great personal cost. It requires trying to make some major adjustments to your work-life balance, and that's not easy. There was a time that you thought you had figured everything out; probably now you'll be wondering how you ever thought that. But, as we both know, life doesn't always turn out as we expected.

Members of my family and I were all called on to help my mother, who had metastatic cancer that had been misdiagnosed. For five years, she suffered in pain, believing what her doctor told her, and that was that she had sciatic nerve discomfort. He prescribed medication that failed to work, and the reason he prescribed that medication was that he was frightened that she might become addicted. He had worked for years in an addictions clinic. Our mother had a deadly diagnosis with no hope for a cure, and he was worried that she would become addicted. How do you worry about addiction with a dying person?

As a result of his experience, he refused to prescribe the pain-relieving medication that she needed. For the years when she was under his care, he never made a referral for more sophisticated testing or imaging. In both respects, he failed my mother, and it proved to be a deadly mistake.

When I persuaded her to go to a different physician, she received the correct diagnosis, but it was too late for any treatment that would save her. At this point, she was no longer able to walk and was confined to her bed for most of the day.

One of my older sisters then proceeded to outline how each of us would take turns caring for her in her home. She made a spreadsheet with our names, the time we were to be there, and which day of the week we were assigned for the entire night. The sheet also listed the medications to administer and other necessary medical provisions. I can't tell you how many times, while on an overnight shift with my mother, I prayed she would slip quietly into that eternal sleep that would give her peace. Did I feel awful when I had that thought? Of course I did, but it also was out of love for her and her life of incredible devotion to all of us.

It was an extremely painful, stressful, and unpredictable time for us, and it lasted for five months. She went through one major operation where the surgeon said, "*The surgery won't save her life, but it will decrease her pain.*" It was all we could hope for, and we agreed. Before the surgery, lying on the gurney, she told each of us that she loved us. After the surgery, we brought her home again because we wanted to care for her there, not in a hospital, where she would be just one of many patients.

Of course, pain medications were finally ordered by an empathic oncologist, but to get the prescription filled was another almost insurmountable task. **No pharmacy would fill it** because it contained one ingredient they refused to carry: cocaine. The pharmacists told me that if they carried cocaine, they would be victimized by repeated robberies. Frantically, we called pharmacy after pharmacy and received the same message that they couldn't or wouldn't do it.

The medication was, at that time, called Brompton's mixture and was a formula from the original hospice programs in Great Britain. After all of those futile attempts, through the intervention of a coworker who knew a pharmacist, we filled the prescription once. The difficulty of having the prescription filled and our discussions with the oncologist moved him to instruct the hospital pharmacy to provide it. They prepared it for us at a fraction of the cost.

I was the designated person to drive to the hospital to pick up the two bottles of liquid. I transported them through a dangerous part of town to bring them to my mother's home. We used only half of one bottle before my mother lapsed into a coma and was transported to the hospital. In that hospital room, the five of us sat with her through the night before she died.

I had been one of the five who cared for her. None of us had any nursing training, but we were required to do many of the tasks that are normally performed by skilled nurses. Each of us learned what to do and provided all that was needed.

Five months seems like a very short time for so many people who are caregivers who will have to care for years, not months. But no matter how long or short the time, it is brutally draining and emotionally demanding. I couldn't know that years later, in my professional training, I would be traveling across the United States as a clinical monitor for a new medication to treat Alzheimer's disease. During that time, I met many caregivers and saw the frustration, the bewilderment and the price they were all paying to care for someone they loved.

I remember the couple in their middle 60s, where the woman kept firing their help because she was convinced they were stealing from her. The situation became so serious that she insisted he install additional burglar and security alarms on the home. At the point when I saw them, they had already installed three of them. In fact, she didn't remember where she put things. Then there was the woman who traveled by car for several hours with her husband and kept turning the radio on and off. The drive was three times as long because they had to keep stopping.

One of the most curious patients in the protocol was a dentist who demanded that his wife remove the patients from their living room. The living room was empty, and he was having visual hallucinations.

Another older woman in her 80s kept insisting she wanted to go home to visit her mother. She was similar to a man who told his wife, each evening, that he had to go home because his parents were expecting him. They had been married for over 50 years, and now he was trying to eat paper clips and thumbtacks and anything he could find in the kitchen. He couldn't tell what was edible and what wasn't. If he walked into the hallway in their apartment building, he couldn't remember how to get back home. They'd already found him locked in a stairwell on the 16th floor of their building. His wife was beside herself and didn't know what to do because they had no relatives nearby and no children.

My mother accused us of serving her spoiled or poisoned food. Even when we presented her with her favorite foods and a special cake from a gourmet shop she had always adored, she declared it spoiled. Cancer, we now know, affects people's ability to taste, and that was happening to my mother. But we were being accused of trying to hurt her.

The most startling instance of cognitive impairment was when a man who had been an engineer slipped rapidly into Alzheimer's and became paranoid. His wife found him in the basement sharpening bayonets to defend them from an unknown threat. He never said who or what the threat was. He just knew they were in danger, and he had to protect them.

Once again, caregivers were in my life, and I wanted to help all of them. It became possible when I could write this book to reach out to all of those who are caregiving now.

One thing to remember here is that you are the caregiver of YOU. Never forget that as you go through this book and these exercises. Care for yourself. Time and time again, you're going to see that reminder throughout this book, and occasionally or frequently, you will want to dismiss it. **Don't dismiss it. It's too important.**

Right now, are you feeling a little resentful, angry, or drained? All of those feelings are expected and normal, so don't ever put yourself down. This is not the normal situation you would be in. You've been brought into a world that presents challenges that once were unimaginable. You've been asked to extend yourself beyond anything reasonable, and you're doing it. It doesn't matter how long you've been doing it; you've now reached a point where you are seeking help, and that's a good thing.

Some days, you probably wanted to cry, or you wanted to scream, or, like the woman I detail later in this book, you have been concerned that you might strike out. Yes, you felt all of those things, but you will learn how you can get yourself under control to benefit you and the one for whom you care. Crying isn't a bad thing, and it doesn't show a lack of strength or resilience. It's a natural process that allows us to release some of those emotions. Do it if you want, and don't be ashamed. You will cry. Do you know what the famous writer Charlotte Brontë said about crying? *"Crying doesn't indicate that you are weak. Since birth, it has always been a sign that you are alive."*

Now is not the time to put yourself down, but it is a time to get the help that you deserve, and it's here. Yes, it's here for you, and you will find things that make this journey a bit more manageable. I know "manageable" is a word that may make you smile because it seems so simple. We know it's not simple, and we know that because all the people that have been going down this path are telling us how demanding the journey has been for them. It is demanding for you, too. I found it, as my sisters did, to be incredibly draining, emotionally and physically. Some of us, in fact, had to drive over an hour before we got to my mother's home, and then we would be met with more of the unexpected.

The Unseen Army of Caregivers

Across the United States alone, more than 53 million people *provide unpaid care to family members or friends*. This number continues to rise as our population ages and advances in medical care enable people to live longer with chronic conditions. Globally, *caregiving touches hundreds of millions of lives* in every community. We are, and various sources have indicated, in the throes of a silver tsunami in terms of an increasing elderly population. But beyond older adults, there is a large and increasing number of individuals with disabilities, both adults and children, who will require our ongoing care. The question becomes: *who will care for the caregivers?*

Caregivers come from every background and walk of life. Some provide full-time care in their homes, while others coordinate care from a distance or balance caregiving with a full work schedule. Many do this work quietly, without formal training, yet with enormous dedication and love.

The Hidden Costs of Caregiving

While caregiving can be deeply rewarding, it often comes with hidden emotional and physical tolls. The chronic stress, interrupted sleep, and constant vigilance can lead to burnout, depression, and health problems. We know that stress in our lives without the responsibility as a caregiver has a great impact on our physical and mental health, so here we see a doubling up of our stress level. It is not uncommon for caregivers to put their own needs last, believing that *their duty is simply part of the role.*

This "always giving" mindset is both a testament to your love and a dangerous path if left unchecked. The truth is, to care effectively for others, **you must care for yourself**. Being a caregiver is not a luxury or indulgence—it's essential. But being a caregiver also requires that you care for yourself, even though that is going to initially appear to be selfish. It is not.

Why This Book Matters

When You Can't Pour From an Empty Cup: CBT Skills for Exhausted Caregivers is designed with you in mind—the overwhelmed, the exhausted, the guilt-ridden, and the *often overlooked caregiver*. This book offers practical, research-based tools grounded in Cognitive Behavioral Therapy (CBT) that can help you:

- Recognize the early signs of burnout and emotional exhaustion.

- Untangle unhelpful thoughts like guilt and perfectionism.

- Reclaim joy through simple, doable activities.

- Face and process difficult emotions like anger and resentment.

- Reduce catastrophic thinking during crisis moments.

- Set healthy boundaries without guilt or shame.

- Build an emotional first-aid kit to weather tough days.

- Reinvent your identity beyond caregiving to nurture yourself.

These skills are not simply about surviving caregiving—they're about learning to thrive within it. I know that thrive may seem a bit odd in a situation like this, but we need to consider that our lives must be attended to as well. Thriving is part of what you need to consider, and doing so needs to be discussed, also. Yes, you matter, and you are appreciated by others, so now we are going to help you appreciate yourself.

Why CBT?

First, let's clarify one point. This is not a book of therapy but a book that uses the therapeutic techniques you can bring into your life and use personally. We do this because cognitive behavioral therapy (CBT) is one of the most effective, evidence-based approaches for managing stress, anxiety, and depression. It focuses on the connections between our thoughts, feelings, and behaviors and offers practical techniques to reshape unhelpful patterns. It provides a real-time approach to understanding and altering your own and others' behaviors.

Unlike therapies that delve deeply into the past, CBT equips you with **tools you can use right now** to improve your day-to-day life. It's accessible, flexible, and adaptable to the unique challenges of caregiving. So, don't think we are going to begin exploring things like "unconscious conflict" or anything other than your daily experiences and the way you relate to them currently.

A Compassionate Approach

This book approaches caregiving with deep compassion and respect. *There is no one "right" way to care for someone*, and there is *no expectation that you will be perfect*. Instead, this book honors your humanity—your strengths, your struggles, and your need for kindness, especially from yourself.

You will find stories from real caregivers, such as mine, who have faced similar challenges, along with exercises and reflections designed to help you engage actively with the material. You can work through this book *at your own pace*, revisiting chapters or exercises whenever you need a boost.

A Lifeline for the Journey

Caregiving is not a quick sprint—it's often a marathon with unexpected twists and turns. You will have days filled with hope and connection and days heavy with exhaustion and doubt. This book is *a lifeline you can return to* in all those moments.

Remember, the tools you develop here don't just benefit you. When you are cared for, you can care better. When you nurture your well-being, your loved one benefits too.

I was reminded here about a woman who worked at the same hospital where I was several decades ago. One day, at lunch, she cried as she talked about her mother's spiral into dementia. The two of them lived alone in a large home, and none of the other family members ever asked if they could help, came over to give her some time for herself, or in any way contributed.

She was becoming more and more aware that she could not handle her mother's disability, and her anger was increasing. "*Last night*," she told me, "*I almost hit her*." As she said this, the tears gushed from her eyes, and I knew she needed help, and it needed to be from outside the family. After that, I found a local organization that stepped in and provided the daycare, the meals, and the respite for this woman and her mother. Eventually, her mother was admitted to a dementia care facility, and the woman felt relieved. It was only then that her family realized how blindsided they had been to her and their mother's needs.

What to Expect

Each chapter focuses on a *common caregiving challenge* and offers CBT-based strategies paired with guided exercises. You can choose the chapters that most align with your current situation instead of reading them all at once.

At the end of the book, you'll find a library of worksheets and tools you can use anytime. These resources are designed to be simple, practical, and adaptable to your needs. Also, I don't believe in jargon or fancy mumbo-jumbo. I believe in dealing with what is best and then going forward. It involves taking incremental steps on a journey you might not have previously imagined.

A Final Thought Before We Begin

Choosing to care for someone else is one of the most profound expressions of love. It is a gift, but it is also a heavy responsibility that can stretch you in ways you never thought. Expect to encounter emotions that may not align with your typical functioning style. *Caregiving is a novel experience for most of us*, and you were walking through the woods on a poorly defined path until you picked up this book.

My book invites you to hold both the gift of giving and the weight with grace and courage. I encourage you to honor your dedication while nurturing your heart.

You deserve to be whole—to be strong, joyful, and supported—throughout your caregiving journey and beyond.

Now that you've read everything in this introduction, I want you to do something for yourself: **sit down**. Yes, sit down and keep the book in your hands. This work is not something to rush through, and it's not something that will not, in some way, be enjoyable. I want you to *enjoy the journey of discovery*. This approach is the only way that all of this material can become a part of you and your behavior.

Ultimately, your success will depend on your behavior and how you think about it. Do I think you're going to be successful? Of course I do. I have faith in anybody who has the wish to change and the courage to pick up a book that helps them do so. Purchasing a book that guides you to transform yourself is a brave act. For me, it's an act of humility that you should prize as one of your best qualities. As a cherished university professor once told our class, "*You are my students, and you will be my students for the rest of your life. If you need me, I will be here."* I will try to always offer you helpful books and articles, even if you aren't my student or my patient.

Let's begin.

Chapter 1: Spotting Burnout Before It Breaks You

Caregiving typically *begins with a belief that it will become a loving experience* that draws you closer to your loved one. However, the ongoing demands of caregiving, including persistent alertness and mental exhaustion, gradually erode the strength of even the most strong-willed individuals.

Your previous willingness to perform tasks now feels as burdensome as wading through thick liquid. Your emotions become sharper with the person you care for, which triggers *immediate feelings of guilt and shame*. A faint inner voice may begin to indicate that your personality has changed significantly. You begin to question yourself and your abilities, and it is an unsettling time for you and the person you care for.

Burnout represents more than simply feeling exhausted. Long-term exposure to excessive stress leads to this experience, which results in emotional and mental depletion together with physical exhaustion. You will experience emptiness alongside detachment, which prevents you from managing everyday requirements. Your sense of self may feel as though it has vanished completely, and you feel like you are just going through the motions or have vanished into nothingness.

Adult caregivers who care for aging parents or partners with health issues experience burnout as a powerful destructive force. Severe burnout symptoms *affect more than one-third of adult caregivers* (37 percent). They experience mental fog that makes decisions impossible, emotional numbness during critical moments, and crushing exhaustion that sleep can't ease.

The prevalence of burnout among child caregivers remains lower than those who are caregivers for adults, with 22 percent of mothers and 19 percent of fathers showing high burnout symptoms. Statistics demonstrate the actual challenge you currently face while maintaining your own stability as you care for others. *No one can escape burnout*, and that's why everyone must know its symptoms and how to deal with it.

Stress is a part of our lives, and, as you begin this book, it may be helpful for you to do a simple evaluation with a well-known adjustment scale, the **Holmes & Rahe Life Change Index**. This is *not to be used as a clinical scale for evaluation of any mental health disorders* but rather as a simple look at where your stress might be coming from. Once you have this in hand, you can then begin to take some steps to counter that. Here's the URL where you can download the scale to your computer: https://socialwork.buffalo.edu (self-care kit).

One additional note is called for here. There is no one who is free from stress because stress, which is simply a change of an emotional state, *comes from the good things happening in our lives as well as the bad ones*. So everyone will have some indication, as shown by a number, of their stress level.

Stress indicator numbers go from less than 150 to over 300. If your stress indicator falls within the 300 range, you may need to seek assistance from a healthcare professional. You can print out the scale, circle the items that fit with your situation, and add up all of the values for each of those items to get your total score. It's a good way to keep track of things, and it's a good reminder that maybe you need to kick back a bit and take it easy or have a serious conversation with someone, perhaps your boss, your family or your neighbors.

Let's also think about how your stress response may have developed. New research has indicated that pregnant women who undergo a great deal of stress transfer that stress to the fetus. The child is then born with a different sensitivity to stress than another child, whose mother may have had much less stress. In this way, stress sensitivity is transferred biologically and not environmentally by seeing your mother's responses to stress. We used to think it was genetic or that we had learned it, but now we have a new perspective on it.

Samantha's Story

Samantha cared for her mother, who suffered from dementia, over the past three years. She initially felt proud and strong because she managed to handle her responsibilities at work as well as care for her family. But slowly, things began to shift. She stopped attending her weekly yoga classes. Friendships were being neglected, and she no longer saw her friends for a weekly lunch at a local restaurant. Home confinement had trapped her, leading to the development of resentment toward her siblings for providing no assistance. Her extended family was feeling disconnected from her, the woman with whom they had always enjoyed family get-togethers.

In the morning, she discovered she hadn't experienced laughter or any emotions for an unknown period of time. Her emotions had turned robotic while she became irritable, and her sadness reached a deep, emotional level. Samantha's burnout caught up with her without her noticing until the point when it consumed her completely. But that's how burnout works, and it is like a thief in the night that is going to steal your joy and make life more difficult each day.

Recognizing Early Warning Signs

Identifying burnout signs during their early stages serves as the key strategy for *preventing complete burnout*. The following signs should be watched for:

- Feeling cynical or disconnected from the person you care for

- Frequent headaches, stomach problems, or other physical complaints

- Increased irritability or emotional outbursts

- Withdrawal from friends, hobbies, or activities you once enjoyed

- Trouble sleeping or excessive sleeping

- Feeling like you're on an emotional coaster

- Constant fatigue that doesn't improve with rest

You might think, "*I just need a good night's sleep,*" or "*Once this busy week is over, I'll feel better.*" A prolonged presence of these feelings indicates to your body and mind that you should **take immediate action**. One thing to remember is that you may not feel all of these things all at once, but you may want to begin checking some of them off. If you feel this way, burnout is starting, but it can take a while.

Why Caregivers Ignore the Signs

Caregivers frequently dismiss help requests because they believe it demonstrates weakness along with failure. Self-sacrifice combined with endless devotion becomes socially validated, even though *no one investigates its impact on caregivers*. You may think self-care is selfish, yet the reality shows that neglecting your needs benefits no one in the future.

Guided Exercise: Burnout Early Warning Checklist

Take a moment to assess your current mental state with complete honesty. Keep a small notebook handy so that you can write down each symptom you identify within yourself.

___I feel exhausted most of the time, even after sleeping. How many hours of sleep did you get last night?

___ I've lost interest in activities I used to enjoy. When did this happen?

___ I feel increasingly irritable or angry.

___ I experience frequent physical complaints (headaches, stomachaches, etc.). Have you had a medical checkup recently?

___ I feel detached or disconnected from others.

___ I feel like I'm on edge or waiting for something bad to happen.

___ I have trouble concentrating or making decisions.

___ I feel guilty for taking breaks or saying no.

Please review the items you have checked after completing the list. The purpose of this exercise is to provide an honest picture of your current state without causing feelings of self-reproach. These are simply points to be aware of in your ongoing quest to help yourself as an overburdened caregiver.

Next Steps

Several checked items indicate you need to implement immediate changes at this point. Delay is not your friend, and if you feel reluctant to reach out, that is a normal reaction to your situation. Many people who are caregivers feel they should be able to handle this totally on their own, but that is self-deception that is injurious to you. *Help yourself now* and reach out to a support group or consult with a mental health professional and, in addition, seek help from your family and friends. There is no shame in asking for help, especially in a caregiving situation.

Often, people or organizations are there to help you, but you don't know it, or, as I've said, you feel reluctant to reach out. I know because our family felt the same way. We only found out about hospice programs, in which my mother was finally involved, after I, unexpectedly, was asked to write a book review on hospice programs in the United States. If that book had not come across my desk, what would have happened to our family? Undoubtedly, it would have been a worse tragedy.

Why hadn't we been referred to any of these programs? Part of the problem was that my mother's primary care physician didn't know about them, hadn't read about them, and they were not widely opening in the United States at that time. In fact, even the word "hospice" was new to us and had to be explained. Now, hospice care is a common service available throughout the world. And we know that part of the service that is offered is to relieve caregivers for a bit of time away from their responsibilities in order to revive themselves.

Your health represents the base that enables you to continue caring for others. Your own well-being stands as the essential support that enhances your capability to serve your loved one and yourself.

Chapter 2: Untangling Guilt and Perfectionism

Caregivers typically bear two unnoticeable weights that come in the form of **guilt and perfectionism**. The constant presence of these burdens makes them so normal that you fail to identify the added weight you carry through your daily lives. Let's explore this a little bit more and see what's happening and what can be changed.

Guilt speaks in your mind through whispers that tell you to extend your efforts. The moment you try to rest for a few minutes, your mind tells you that you are being lazy. A single minor mistake triggers perfectionism, which labels you as someone who disappoints the person you care about. Does perfection really exist in our world? No, it doesn't, and anyone seeking to be perfect has set themselves up for a major disappointment or to constantly feel inadequate.

Perfectionism's harsh inner voice demands flawless execution of all tasks. It's the expectations that demand that you maintain patience and readiness while remaining strong all the time. Any misstep you make triggers an overwhelming sense of total failure. As you might begin to see here, you don't need to be perfect, and you don't need to be strong all the time. We are fallible human beings, and we will do some things well and other things not so well. But that's the nature of being a human being.

Anna's Story

Anna devoted herself to caring for her husband following his stroke. Not only had her husband suffered a major stroke, he was now confined to bed unless an assistant was brought in to help place him in a special wheelchair. There were other medical procedures that also required tubing and changing and specialized fluids that needed to be administered. Anna had done none of this type of work, and she was distressed and felt she couldn't handle it. She managed his therapy sessions while handling his medications and his bathing needs, along with preparing the placement of nutritional fluids via a port in his stomach. She performed every task without support because she felt it was her responsibility to manage everything on her own. Not for a moment did Anna consider that she had never had any nursing training or that medical procedures were beyond her ability.

The development of a pressure sore on her husband brought tremendous distress to Anna. Despite the doctor's reassurances about the typical nature of his condition and her lack of responsibility for it, she could not shake off the feeling of self-blame. She repeated to herself without stopping, "*A better caregiver would prevent this mistake from happening.*"

The demands of Anna's perfectionism stopped her from seeking assistance from her adult children. She worried they would consider her incapable. Her belief pushed her into deeper exhaustion and created feelings of resentment.

Breaking the "Should" Cycle

Cognitive behavioral therapy skills help patients to both test and rewrite their unproductive mental patterns. Instead of repeating the phrase "*I should do everything perfectly*" you should tell yourself, "*I am doing the best I can with what I have available today.*" Remember that each day is not only a new day but also a learning opportunity that will hone your skills and enable you to be more proficient in what is needed. It's not a class you sought to attend, but you are a student now.

Record your "should" statements for better analysis through this helpful exercise. For each one, ask:

• Is this belief realistic? How did you come to that belief?

• Where did this expectation come from? Did someone tell you this or did you come up with it yourself?

• Would I say this to a dear friend in the same situation? OK, what would you say to a dear friend?

Examples of Reframed Thoughts

The phrase "*I should never lose my patience*" should be replaced with "*Everyone loses patience sometimes. I can apologize and move forward.*" In mental health situations, we generally tell people that when something is causing you to lose patience with someone, what you do is step back out of the situation and take a few minutes' break. It's these breaks that enable you to refocus and rethink what's going on. Use that technique whenever you begin to feel this way.

The statement "*I should be able to do this alone*" should be rewritten as "*Getting assistance does not indicate weakness since it proves my human nature.*" Why should you go it alone? Is there something wrong with getting help with something? If you're thinking that way, you're being too hard on yourself. Loosen up and allow yourself what you need when you need it.

Guided Exercise: Compassionate Caregiver Mantra

Choose a personal mantra that feels right to you. Do them as often as you feel you need, and don't hesitate whenever you are beginning to question yourself. These examples *serve as motivation* for your personal development:

- *"I am enough, as I am today."*
- *"Taking care of myself helps me care for others."*
- *"I deserve compassion, too."*

Write down your chosen mantra, then position it in places you visit frequently, such as the bathroom mirror, the fridge, or your bedside table. Verbalize your mantra to yourself daily. While we took care of our mother, we posted everything on the refrigerator door because that's where everyone saw it numerous times every day. There was no forgetting anything once it was on that refrigerator door.

Requesting Help Never Indicates Defeat

The most powerful demonstration of strength emerges when we recognize our need for help. Make a list of assignments that you can distribute to others. You could ask your neighbor to buy your groceries while your friend watches your loved one so you can take a break. People are there for you. Believe me. Once you begin to reach out, you will see that help exist.

When you share responsibilities with others, it does not reduce your love or commitment to care for them, but helps maintain it. The ability to help others depends on having enough content in your own emotional reservoir since you cannot fill another person's needs from an empty glass. That's right, the empty glass benefits no one.

Permission to Be Human

Our relentless pursuit of perfection and self-judgment creates an endless pattern that perfectionism keeps us trapped within. Recognizing our humanity, accepting mistakes, resting, and experiencing both happiness and sadness all contribute to a stronger source of resilience. Each step you take is beneficial for you and the person for whom you care.

Your "perfect" caregiving abilities do not determine your ability to give wonderful care to others. The genuine and loving nature of your care emerges precisely from your human imperfections.

Chapter 3: Reclaiming Joy Through Behavioral Activation

The endless list of responsibilities in a caregiver's life tends to transform into a never-ending task list. The passing days create confusion, while the enjoyable pursuits that brought you happiness disappear completely. You find yourself wondering without any awareness of what used to bring you pleasure.

Losing joy represents a fundamental reason why caregivers experience feelings of emptiness and detachment. Behavioral Activation stands as a vital CBT technique that helps people regain their spark of joy.

The Power of Small Pleasures

The foundation of Behavioral Activation rests on the fundamental principle that people *take action before experiencing emotions*. The method involves beginning with a pleasant activity before positive emotions develop naturally. This way, it's essentially a push to engage in some behavior because you know that the end result will be positive.

Several tiny actions prove that they can penetrate the mental haze that affects you. Your connection to your forgotten identity can begin with short activities like sunlit walks while singing favorite songs or socializing with previous friends. Did you know that even humming can be a spirit-lifting activity?

Most people don't know about that research, but it has shown that, just like in the Disney movie where Cinderella is humming and singing while doing her chores, it can help you, too. And you are not in a Disney movie. Yes, you can laugh as you read that, and it's a good thing, too. While I'm on the subject, researchers have shown that laughing lifts our mood and exercises our entire body, so we do a couple of good things at one time whenever we laugh. Take the opportunity and laugh whenever you can. It can be a lifesaver in terms of mental health. I've known people who made it a practice to keep comedy films on their computers so that they could sit down and have a laugh every once in a while. As long as they could laugh at any part of the film, it didn't matter how many times they'd seen it. To them, it was a lifesaver.

Marcus's Story

While caring for his injured brother, Marcus provided support. Before starting caregiving, Marcus used to prepare complicated dinners as a hobby. He completely stopped cooking after his responsibilities expanded. The kitchen experiments he yearned for emerged as his top desire, yet he felt that such activities were now out of reach. No, Marcus was going to deny himself that joy because he believed that while his brother was being cared for, he should not be enjoying anything.

The counselor helped Marcus develop a strategy that involved starting with small steps. During his dinner preparation, he devoted fifteen minutes to preparing a basic pasta dish with fresh herbs. His experience of chopping and smelling and tasting brought back feelings of peaceful joy, which he had not experienced in many years. It was simple and only involved chopping herbs, but it was emotionally fulfilling.

A single cooking session marked the beginning of his weekly practice, which he treated as his special time. The weekly cooking practice became something he eagerly expected, as it helped him build patience and energy throughout his caregiving responsibilities. Cooking is not merely a simple preparation of meals; it is, in fact, a gift of health for everyone who enjoys the food.

Guided Exercise: Joyful Activities Menu

Create a new sheet of paper with *My Joyful Activities Menu written* at the top of the page. The paper should contain three distinct sections, which follow below:

1. Quick joys (5–10 minutes): Examples—stepping outside to breathe fresh air, listening to a favorite song, savoring a cup of tea. These are things that take a little time, but even a breath of fresh air has rejuvenated possibilities.

2. Moderate Joys (30–60 minutes): Examples—meeting a friend for coffee, working on a hobby, going for a short hike. It's not so much the breaks in time as it is being in a new situation or being "freed" from the caregiving for a bit.

3. Big Joys (a few hours or a day): Examples—visiting a museum, taking a day trip to the beach, attending a workshop. For this, obviously, you will need someone who will pick up the responsibilities for you for that day or those hours. Yes, you can find someone who will

do this, so begin your search and make a list of them and their available days, times and phone numbers.

Select a brief, joyful activity that you can add to your schedule during this week. Write this down in your schedule like any other critical caregiving responsibility because it holds the same importance. You've made the schedule, I know, so be sure to fill in the space for your joyful activity, and don't fail to engage in it. If you want to see that as a mandate from me, go right ahead.

Scheduling Joy Without Guilt

You might feel hesitant or even selfish for making time for these activities. The process of filling your emotional tanks serves as an **essential requirement** instead of an optional treat. The practice of participating in joyful activities builds up your ability to present yourself with patience and kindness and presence. Guilt be gone, and let the fun come on.

Start Small, Celebrate Often

The power of small beginnings shouldn't be ignored. You don't need to make drastic changes to your life in one night. The process of adding small joyful moments is like adding water to a dry sponge, which helps you grow stronger and more robust with each drop. What happens to a sponge if you let it dry out? Right, it becomes brittle and stiff, and you don't want to use it anymore. Keep your resilience going, and don't become stiff like that old sponge.

Acknowledge every attempt regardless of its magnitude. Your growing awareness of particular activities you miss proves that you are reconnecting with your personal needs and desires.

A Living List

Your **Joyful Activities: The menu** exists to change as you wish. Your *Joyful Activities Menu is not static*. Your activities will transform as you grow and develop. The path of discovery might lead you to discover new interests or revive forgotten activities that seemed lost forever. This list, as always, must stay visible to you so you can refer to it whenever feelings of disconnection from yourself arise. When that happens, head for that menu and see what you might be able to do at that time. It's your life preserver if you think the ship might be going down, and that's why it's there for you. Yes, if you want, think of this list as your little "floaties" that kids use when they're first learning to swim. You are going to swim, and this is the way to do it.

Chapter 4: Facing Resentment and Unspoken Anger

Caregivers commonly hide their feelings of anger from others. Revealing this type of emotion seems both improper and embarrassing to you. You may reason that you should not feel frustrated because you need to take care of someone. The suppression of these emotions allows you to persist rather than disappear.

I don't think that allowing others to know that you are feeling angry is a bad thing. Everyone expects the normal display of emotions, given any situation they happen to be experiencing at that moment. If anger is appropriate because of what's happening, then you feel angry. There's nothing wrong with that. How you express the anger is what you need to consider how you express your anger. Unfortunately, some caregivers vent their anger on the person they are providing care to, and the result is a distressing situation for all.

I knew a woman who owned a large piece of property in a major town where she had a two-family house. Her parents died, leaving her to care for a sister with a mental disorder and limited vision. What was she going to do? Her choice was not a favorable one, and she put her sister into a single room in one of the large homes that she owned.

She left the sister alone for hours during the day, providing her with only breakfast and dinner at night. That was the only interaction she had with anyone while she lived there. The woman lived in that room for at least two years until her sister married and sold the house and moved away, taking her sister with her. I hope the next situation was better for that poor sister who was alone for so long, but I don't know.

Suppressing these angry emotions allows them to continue growing until they reach a critical point. The stored feelings manifest as irritability toward family members or emotional numbness and random outbursts of crying. Consider the actions that the sister took against her younger sister, who is impaired. The situation was truly tragic, and I don't believe her parents ever expected her to react in that way.

Tom's Story

After his father suffered a major stroke, Tom took responsibility for his father's care. Tom's heart broke upon witnessing his independent and proud father's decline, prompting him to resign his job and move into his father's house. At first, he assured himself he felt privileged to provide assistance.

But the prolonged months of care led Tom to experience an intense sense of confinement. Most evenings he spent alone since his friends stopped reaching out to him. The sudden desire to help his father, followed by intense feelings of shame and guilt, made him angry at himself. He maintained substantial resentment, which he refused to consider because he had never given himself permission to do so.

The ABCs of Understanding Your Anger

Cognitive Behavioral Therapy teaches people to use the ABC model for better emotional understanding.

The **activating event (A)** represents the triggering event that produces anger or resentment.

Belief (B) stands for the internal dialogue about the situation.

The emotional response and **physical actions of C** result from these situations.

Example:

A relative gives you negative feedback about how you assisted them with dressing.

1. The criticism I receive *makes me feel helpless* because I fail at everything I try to do. I'm a terrible caregiver.

2. The way *you feel defeated and angry* makes you withdraw emotionally.

3. The emotional pain stems from your beliefs about the situation rather than the event itself. *Changing your beliefs* will lead to changes in your emotional responses.

This process of *reframing beliefs* means you should replace *"I must always be perfect and patient"* with *"I am doing my best in a very difficult situation, and that is enough."* It is enough. It's not good for you or the person you care for to think you should be doing more without any special training or knowledge.

The process will not eliminate all your anger, but it will help you observe it without self-criticism. Always see if reframing is possible in any situation. Believe me, there will be situations that will arise, and you will be thankful that you can reframe them.

Guided Exercise: ABC Worksheet

Use a recent incident that triggered resentment or frustration within you.

1. Write down the complete details of what happened (Acti-

vating Event)?

2. What thought ran through your mind (Belief)?

3. How did you feel and react (Consequence)?

Then ask:

- *Is my belief entirely accurate? Always question your thoughts and how they may have been influenced by your beliefs.*

- Where does the supporting and opposing evidence for your belief exist?

- A different perspective about this situation could be more balanced.

Allow Yourself to Experience Emotions

You have permission to experience anger as an emotion. You have the right to yearn for a respite. Your human nature expresses itself through these feelings, which do not reduce your love for this person. Remember what I said about my time at night while caring for my mother? What was my wish? Did it mean I loved her any less? No, it didn't.

Finding Healthy Outlets

The following methods provide you with *safe ways to express your anger*:

- Writing in a private journal

- A conversation with either a trusted friend or therapist.

- Physical movement (walking briskly, punching a pillow, dancing it out). Dancing is a great way to deal with anger because it freezes your body physically, and when you do it to music, you also give your mind a rest. Music is very soothing, even if it's the type of music one woman I knew liked—John Philip Sousa marches. Yes, she marched around the house whenever she became upset with anger, and it helped.

- Artistic expressions through music and other forms of creativity. Any type of artistic activity can be helpful, including painting, drawing, writing, working with clay or even small plants in your home. I know one man who has found that growing small bonsai trees is a wonderful relief from his daily stress. Another woman I knew used poetry writing as her outlet.

Hiding your emotions results in negative effects on both your mental and physical state. It's a sure thing that using healthy outlets to express your anger allows you to maintain your energy while developing authentic care for your loved one instead of harboring hidden resentment.

The Gift of Honesty

Caregivers who face and process their anger openly usually experience a feeling of relief from a mental burden that they have placed on themselves. The practice of honesty produces genuine relationships between yourself and the person you support as well as between you and your authentic self.

Love does not determine whether you experience resentment. The prolonged disregard of your personal needs creates this warning sign. The first step to achieving balance and healing requires you to *listen to these feelings.*

Chapter 5: Reducing Catastrophic Thinking in Crisis Moments

Caregivers experience an endless stream of potential negative scenarios. Thoughts that run through their mind are many and troubling. For example, they may think the safety of someone depends on my continuous presence because *I worry they might fall.* Or, it might be, *I worry about giving the wrong medication dosage.* First thing that might bring up more stress is when someone is thinking *The situation is beyond my control when emergencies occur.* All negative, very concerning thoughts.

The mental process of catastrophic thinking involves believing the most disastrous outcome will surely occur, and it seems inevitable.

These protective thoughts produce chronic anxiety, which drains both your mental clarity and your physical power.

Jasmine's Story

After a severe car accident, Jasmine dedicated herself to caring for her teenage daughter. But she experienced fear every time her daughter made a coughing sound because she feared pneumonia and additional hospital visits and even worse outcomes. Every trivial change triggered a total panic attack for her. Daily, she was on alert, waiting for some sign that something terrible was about to happen and she would have to jump in to rescue her daughter. It was a time without rest and of ongoing surveillance.

Jasmine learned CBT skills, which revealed to her that these thoughts functioned as mental narratives she created to stay alert. Her constant state of being watchful led her to remain in a state of fear, along with exhaustion.

Understanding Catastrophic Thinking

The process of catastrophic thinking begins when an initial trigger activates (like a cough or a missed medication) before triggering a series of imagined catastrophic events. Your body fails to recognize imaginary threats from actual threats, which results in your nervous system operating at maximum alert. There is an alarm level of stress, and then the exhaustion kicks in.

Psychologists have studied this type of ongoing stress, and what they have discovered is that it can have very serious physical effects on health. The stress theory of Hans Selye indicated that persistent activation of a constantly high stress level can lead to a breakdown of physiological systems and increase the risk of stress-related illnesses, including *cardiovascular disease, high blood pressure, and ulcers*. In severe cases, exhaustion can even be fatal. Stress, as we now know, damages, our immune system and leaves us prone to all kinds of illnesses. Think about it. If controlling our stress can keep us healthy, then that's the thing to do, correct?

There is another psychologist, Martin Seligman, who looked at how people react in stressful situations. He believed that they may have learned, early in their lives, to be helpless which led to their depression, and they must also now learn how to be active on their behalf.

Catastrophic thinking, in my mind, is a form of learned helplessness. Seligman believed this was the basis for most depression. Of course, now we know that depression is much more complex than a belief system, and it may be caused by a variety of things, including genetic inheritance, medications, or even certain types of physical illnesses.

Take a few minutes out right now and think back to a time when you were possibly a child or young adult living at home. When a situation arose that was particularly upsetting for the family or your parents, how did they deal with it? Remember, your parents are your first teachers. You, as a child or even as a young adult, tended to model your behavior and your thinking after their behavior and beliefs. After all, they're supposed to be the ones who know what to do in any situation. If they didn't know what to do in a situation, what would you have learned at that point?

Yes, you may have learned that you were helpless to do anything, and you were a victim of chance or someone else. We see many people who have had these experiences, but they know now to question and to see that they do have abilities and power that they can use to resolve situations that seem hopeless. All is not lost, unless you lose the belief that you have hope.

The method of CBT enables us to analyze our thoughts methodically so we can take back control of our situation.

The Thought Record Tool

The thought record serves as a systematic tool for testing catastrophic thinking patterns. **This is how it functions**:

1. Situation: What happened? (e.g., *"My loved one skipped breakfast."*)

2. Automatic Thought: What was your immediate worry? (e.g., *"They'll get weak and faint, and I'll have to call an ambulance."*)

3. Evidence For: What supports this thought? (e.g., *"They have fainted before when not eating."*)

4. Evidence Against: What contradicts this thought? (e.g., *"They ate a big dinner last night. They usually eat later on busy mornings."*) Isn't this another way of reframing what has just happened?

5. Alternative Thought: What's a more balanced way to view it? (e.g., *"They might feel a bit tired, but they can eat later and be fine."*)

6. Outcome: How do you feel now? You've gone over all the possibilities for and against, and now you've come to some reasonable resolution.

Guided Exercise: Crisis Calm Plan & Thought Record

Make a thought record whenever the "what if" worries start flooding your mind during a crisis. The process helps you view your situation from a fresh perspective outside your automatic fear response.

Develop your own Crisis Calm Plan to use when panic arises. A set of grounding methods exists that you can use to stop panic from growing. Your plan might include:

Deep breathing exercises (inhale for 4 counts, hold for 4, exhale for 6)

You should use the mantra *"I can handle this moment"* as a reminder to help you stay focused.

You should *reach out to a friend* or someone who supports you.

You should *take a walk outside* to breathe some fresh air. Did you know that breathing fresh air is therapeutic? Outdoor, fresh air contains chemicals from vegetation in the area, and they can stimulate your nervous system to calm down. It can, and there's research to show that it is, so it's not just an empty suggestion here. You've got research on your side.

The Power of Repetition

The process of completing thought records can feel exhausting or artificial during the initial stages. Your ability to recognize catastrophic thoughts at an early stage will improve as you practice, and you will learn to stop them from growing out of control. As time passes, you will notice that your body remains calmer and your sleep improves while you are present with the person for whom you care.

Reclaiming Peace

The arrival of crisis situations remains inevitable, yet you can learn to handle them with greater stability. Your ability to handle crises with confidence and resourcefulness and resilience entitles you to experience peace of mind because you understand your capabilities. Unfortunately, too many people don't give themselves credit for having abilities they've never had to use before and in which they now have become proficient.

Catastrophic thoughts function as made-up narratives rather than accurate realities. Your ability to rewrite these thoughts allows you to restore your mental clarity as well as your emotional calmness and your life-force.

Chapter 6: Strengthening Boundaries Without Guilt

Caregivers commonly believe that refusing requests violates the essence of loving someone. The belief states that genuine caregiving requires permanent, selfless devotion to constant availability for others.

This belief system silently damages your physical and mental health and emotional state. Caregiving becomes a path toward burnout and resentment instead of love when boundaries are not established.

Why Boundaries Matter

Relationships find protection through boundaries, which act as bridges instead of walls to block others. Your establishment of clear boundaries creates space that enables you to rest while also allowing you to recharge before providing authentic and compassionate care.

Carla's Story

Carla took responsibility for caring for her father when he received his Parkinson's disease diagnosis. She constantly felt obligated to answer every request from her father by staying awake all night while he slept. She gave up her meals to fulfill his needs and refused social invitations because she believed he needed constant attention.

The result? Carla felt invisible in her own life. Her irritability grew toward her father while she developed a strong dislike for each passing day. She discovered through counseling that her fear of being labeled selfish maintained her trapped state. Then, she implemented small boundaries in her daily routine, including thirty-minute walks and allowing a family friend to stay with her father when she went for lunch.

Protecting her time and energy allowed Carla to become more patient and present after she returned.

Common Boundary Myths

- Myth: Saying "no" means I don't care.

Truth: Saying no protects your ability to continue caring.

- Myth: I have to do everything myself.

Truth: Asking for help is a sign of strength, not failure.

- Myth: They will be upset if I set limits.

Truth: Discomfort is normal at first. In the long run, boundaries strengthen trust and respect.

Guided Exercise: Creating Boundary Scripts

Most caregivers refrain from establishing boundaries because they lack the ability to communicate them effectively. A prepared script can help.

1. Identify a scenario where you typically overextend yourself.

2. Develop a polite yet firm written response that you will use for this particular situation.

Examples:

- I will check on you in the next hour, since I can't help you right now.

- I will not extend my work hours today. We need to discuss getting extra support.

- You need to allow me to step away right now so that I can offer better help in the future.

Practice these scripts aloud. The process of practicing these scripts will make you feel more prepared to handle such situations when they occur. If you need a bit of help, practice them in front of a mirror and look at yourself as you say them. Body language is important also, so when you're using your scripts, look at how you stand and what your face looks like. Practice.

Small Steps Lead to Big Shifts

You don't have to overhaul all your boundaries at once. Choose one small limit to set this week. You should celebrate your accomplishments no matter how insignificant they appear. The accumulation of small boundary-setting actions will create a solid base for both self-care and self-respect.

Permission to Prioritize Yourself

The process of scheduling personal needs may feel unusual during the beginning. Each time you uphold your boundaries, you strengthen the conviction that your well-being deserves recognition.

Strong boundaries create a space for you to present yourself with a genuine heart and clear mind to others. When you establish limits with affection, you safeguard both your own health and the person you are taking care of.

Chapter 7: Building Your Emotional First-Aid Kit

The preparations for caregiving emergencies include well-arranged medications and appointment backup systems and a hospital emergency bag. But what about emotional emergencies?

The majority of caregivers fail to prepare for emotional emergencies that suddenly hit them with feelings of being overwhelmed or sad or panicked. The emotional first-aid kit represents your own assembly of personalized tools that help you cope when your emotional resources run out. While not a panacea, this collection offers crucial stability in managing overwhelming emotions.

One area that few caregivers have ever considered is that they experience a special kind of loss, known as *Acquired Non-Death Interpersonal Loss*. What does it mean? The caregiver grieves the old relationship, adapts to a new self, and rebuilds their relationship.

Grief is a part of the caregiving process, too. You are caught between two different realities, the past and the present, and there is *both grief and mental distress* caused by this. For some, this realization may come as a shock, but time has a way of allowing us to rebuild the possible in sometimes seemingly impossible situations. You have strength, and you will build on it, but right now, you might question that ability.

Why You Need an Emotional First-Aid Kit

The unpredictable changes in caregiving bring sudden negative experiences, including bad medical reports, sleepless nights and hurtful comments from family members. During these emotional crises, we use habits that block our feelings instead of providing comfort, which leads us to scroll endlessly, eat excessively and shut down emotionally. These are attempts at self-soothing that are lacking in their ability to provide what we desperately seek. But there are things that you can do.

An emotional first-aid kit functions as a purposeful tool to help you respond to situations with care instead of panicking. A physical reminder exists to demonstrate that your emotional health needs equal attention to the physical health of your loved one.

Michael's Story

Michael took care of his wife during the advanced stages of cancer. The daytime brought him energy, but the night brought on a state of anxiety. He began collecting comforting items such as a playlist of safety songs, an eye pillow with lavender scent and a journal for late-night writings.

The collection he assembled became known to him as his "*night stand kit.*" During difficult evenings, instead of tossing in bed thinking about his worries, he would select these items from his collection. Through time, he understood that these small acts did not remove his grief or worry, *but they helped him* feel less isolated with his emotions.

What Goes Into Your Kit

You should personalize every item in your emotional first-aid kit to reflect your unique nature. Consider including:

- Your comfort kit should contain *soft blankets* together with meaningful *photographs and specific objects* that help you stay present in the moment.

- Include *soothing scents* such as lavender or eucalyptus together with chocolate pieces and a smooth stone for holding purposes.

- *Music or sounds*: A calming *playlist* or nature sounds that soothe your mind. Many of these can be found on the Internet.

- *Written words*: Favorite poems, inspirational quotes, or letters from loved ones. My favorite is: *"If I am not for myself, then who will be for me? If I am but for myself, who am I? And if not now, when?"*

- You can also use the following grounding tools: *Simple breathing exercises and a repeating mantra* like, *"This moment is hard, but I can handle it," and a brief meditation script.*

- The kit should include *contact information for friends and family* members along with online support group details.

Guided Exercise: Create Your Emotional First-Aid Kit

Take a few minutes to reflect:

1. When feeling overwhelmed what things give you comfort?

2. What are the tiny items that make you feel protected and understood and peaceful?

3. A list of people you can contact when feeling alone.

Begin your list and start *collecting these items into a compact box or special carrying bag*. Store it in a reachable spot, such as your bedroom or living room, to grab it whenever you need it most. This is your "go to" bag, and it serves the same purpose as the bags that are used for people who are concerned about natural disasters. In a way, this is a natural disaster, but you will survive this one, and you have the means to do it.

Making It a Ritual

It might seem unusual at first because we lack practical training in self-care. Your emotional first-aid kit becomes a comforting practice each time you use it to remind yourself that you deserve attention, too.

Every time you choose to use your kit, you practice self-compassion. The regular practice of these minor gestures increases your strength so you can handle caregiving challenges instead of succumbing to them.

You Deserve Care, Too

The true essence of caregiving involves sustaining your own human connection as you support another person. Your emotional first-aid kit functions to respect the fragile equilibrium between your own emotional state and the emotional state of your loved one.

Chapter 8: Reinventing Your Identity Beyond Caregiving

The time we spend caregiving can transform into such a significant part of our daily routine that it creates the illusion of *becoming our entire identity*. People who care for others often develop the habit of calling themselves solely caregivers and believing this role encompasses their entire existence. Despite being hidden for a while, your rich and complex identity persists beneath the exhaustion and routine.

Lila's Story

For five years, Lila cared for her aging father. She postponed every dream and interest she had throughout that entire time. The move from her father's home to assisted living left Lila feeling completely without direction. After her father entered assisted living, she suddenly encountered the identity question, which she had not asked herself for many years.

The initial consideration of this question caused her to feel frightened. She worried that her life would become empty without caregiving responsibilities. Over time, she started rediscovering her previous interests, which included painting and volunteering and joining a book club. Through this experience, she rediscovered aspects of her personality that she had thought were lost forever.

Why Reinventing Your Identity Matters

The preservation of your complete personal identity is essential for your health and wellness. Your mental health will benefit from your strong personal identity after caregiving ends, no matter how long the caregiving period lasts.

Maintaining other interests during caregiving activities *creates a stress balance* and maintains your connection to personal growth and purpose and joy.

Writing a Vision Letter to Your Future Self Exercise

Look at yourself through the lens of five years into your future. You have achieved a lifestyle that combines meaningfulness with balance and joy, along with caregiving responsibilities.

Write a letter *to your future self* by following these instructions:

• Your aspirations extend beyond caring for others.

• Make a list of activities you desire to pursue or resume. Allow yourself some latitude here.

• Values that guided your life.

The list includes patience along with creativity and resilience as qualities you wish to develop.

Describe your expectations about how your relationships will change.

Your life contains various sections, and this caregiving chapter stands as an essential but not definitive part of your narrative.

Small Steps to Rediscover Yourself

- Make time to resume activities you stopped doing.

- Start something new that can occupy just a few minutes weekly.

- Take part in a group or enroll in a class that sparks your interest.

- Schedule time for building friendships along with social activities.

- Reflect on your fulfillment sources at regular intervals.

Balancing Roles

You can accept caregiving as a central part of your existence, but there's more to you than that. Your spirit receives nourishment through other roles and interests, which you incorporate into your life to achieve balance.

By setting aside dedicated time for yourself, you will enhance both your personal wellness and bring increased vitality to your caregiving duties. Ask yourself honestly: How much time do you ever set aside for yourself right now? Is there ever any time?

Your Life, Your Story

Your identity remains adaptable while it continues to transform throughout your life. The caregiving experience serves as an essential part of your journey, but it does not represent the complete narrative of your life. In addition to your caregiving duties, you keep your full personhood. Your life deserves to be filled with richness and satisfaction, as you are a complete person with value. But remember that you are the one who must give yourself the freedom that you deserve in a life that you design for the future.

If you don't believe that you deserve to enjoy your life and to spend it on fulfilling activities, no book can convince you otherwise. This book is a small step toward changing that belief, and it is vital to your future self. I hope you take advantage of every opportunity presented here because I sincerely want you to do well.

Our family discovered a new bond that we had not had before caring for my mother. Yes, we benefited from this experience and we will continue to benefit as we reflect on all that we accomplished. We know we did the best we could. Nothing was perfect, but we are human, and perfection is an unwise expectation. **Allow yourself to be human, and allow yourself to live.**

Chap. 9: A New Start Instead of an End: You Deserve Your Wholeness Just as Much as Anyone Else

Caregiving is an extraordinary display of love and sacrifice that requires complete dedication. The role of caregiving stands as one of the most demanding responsibilities, which exhausts the body while creating emotional distress and social separation.

This book has shown you that *self-care represents a necessity rather than selfishness*. You cannot give away what you don't have. Your health is equally important to the person who receives your care.

The CBT tools and exercises you have practiced here are not just techniques; they are also acts of self-compassion. These tools help you uncover the complex feelings of *guilt, exhaustion, and overwhelming emotions*, allowing you to rediscover your inner joy, strength, and resilience.

Remember all the people we've described here and what they confronted in their work. The stories show caregiving doesn't require you to give up your identity. Learning to handle the multiple aspects of love and hardship together with joy and frustration and hope, and grief forms the essence of this experience.

You are not alone on this journey. It's acceptable to ask for assistance while you establish limits and express both anger and sadness. Your human nature reveals itself through these emotions, which do not indicate failure. I've always believed that there is no such thing as failure when you are trying to do something you may not have done before.

What you are doing is learning to do something new, and that's never a failure, no matter how it turns out. Sometimes, you will have to repeat some action several times until you establish a facility in it, and that's learning, too. It's all about learning and love and combining both of them in a way that benefits you and the person for whom you care. **No, there's no failure here.**

Your mental health priorities, combined with the CBT skills from this book, will create a support system for your most challenging times while helping you discover happiness in between. This essential truth should accompany your journey as a caregiver, reminding you that you deserve the same wholeness as everyone else.

Show yourself the same gentle care that you provide to others. Your existence together with your narrative holds equal value.

Appendix: CBT Tools & Worksheets Library

C aregivers can employ these CBT worksheets to get practical support during their most challenging times. Caring for others brings deep meaning, yet this task can cause emotional exhaustion and frustration that eventually lead to self-loss. Through regular or weekly use of these worksheets, caregivers will develop improved thought transformation abilities while creating boundaries and uncovering fundamental requirements and life values.

The ABC Worksheet helps caregivers analyze complex emotions, which primarily comprise anger and resentment. Through this exercise, caregivers can develop improved emotional outcomes by finding the sources of stress.

Through identifying the activating event and its consequences, you can determine the underlying beliefs so a balanced alternative thought can be created. You can build essential emotional control skills through this practice that are necessary for maintaining well-being.

The Thought Record process helps you learn to manage unhelpful negative thought patterns. Evaluating evidence that supports or contradicts your distressing thoughts will reveal alternative realistic perspectives to you. This approach, practiced regularly, leads to decreasing anxiety levels and enables caregivers to better handle their emotional reactions.

Using the Burnout Early Warning Checklist allows you to monitor your mental and physical health to stop reaching burnout points. By recognizing irritability together with withdrawal symptoms and physical discomfort, you can take preventive measures against major burnout through rest and support.

The Joyful Activities Menu works as a basic tool to help you remember you deserve happiness and personal success despite your caregiving responsibilities. A single weekly enjoyable activity creates stronger self-value, which simultaneously reduces emotional exhaustion.

Through the Boundary Scripts and the Emotional First-Aid Kit, you can acquire skills to protect your needs. These scripts, again, help you set boundaries without guilt, and the first-aid kit contains calming items to help you stay centered during stressful moments.

All the worksheets demonstrate the ability to meet personal needs with the same care and kindness that you provide to others. Remember that the worksheets can be reviewed repeatedly to make modifications that function as ongoing tools for strengthening resilience while maintaining personal identity throughout caregiving tasks. The choice to select or change any approach depends on you. **You are in charge here.**

CBT Worksheets for Caregivers

1. **ABC Worksheet**

A   c   t   i   v   a   t   i   n   g

Event:_____

B   e   l   i   e   f   :

_____

Consequence (feelings & actions):_____

Alternative   Balanced

Thought:_____

New   Outcome:

_____

2. Thought Record

Situation: _____

Automatic Thought:

_____

Evidence For:

_____

Evidence Against: _____

Alternative Thought: _____

Outcome (new feelings/behaviors): _____

3. Burnout Early Warning Checklist

Check off any that apply:

___Persistent fatigue

___Loss of interest or pleasure

___Emotional numbness

___Frequent irritability or sadness

___Physical complaints (headaches, stomach issues)

___Trouble sleeping

___Withdrawal from social contact

4. Joyful Activities

Write down activities that bring you joy (big or small):

- _____

- _____

- _____

- _____

Schedule at least one per week.

- _____

5. Boundary Script Examples

- "I understand you need this, but I also need to rest so I can keep helping."

- "I cannot fulfill this request at present, but I will assist you with ___ at a later time."

Your personalized scripts:

- _____

- _____

- _____

6. Emotional First-Aid Kit Planner

List items that comfort and ground you:

- _____

- _____

List emergency supportive contacts:

- _____

- _____

List phrases or reminders to encourage yourself:

- _____

- _____

Suggested Resources and Support Contacts

AARP Caregiving Resources

Phone: N/A (Online resources and local chapter contacts available)

Website: www.aarp.org/caregiving/

Alzheimer's Association

Phone: (800) 272-3900 (24/7 Helpline) Website: www.alz.org

Caregiver Action Network

Phone: (855) 227-3640 (Help Desk) Website: www.caregiveraction.

org

Eldercare Locator

Phone: (800) 677-1116 Website: eldercare.acl.gov

Family Caregiver Alliance

Phone: Contact information varies by state/region (see website for local contacts) Website: www.caregiver.org

National Alliance for Caregiving

Phone: Contact information available through the website. Website: www.caregiving.org

VA Caregiver Support Program

Phone: (855) 260-3274 (Caregiver Support Line) Website: www.caregiver.va.gov

Well Spouse Association

Phone: (800) 838-0879 (toll-free) or (732) 577-8899 Website: wellspouse.org

These organizations provide various forms of support

Support groups and peer connections: Caregiver Action Network Educational resources and training: VA Caregiver Support ProgramVA Caregiver Support Program

Information and referral services to local resources: Eldercare Locator, connecting you to services for older adults and families–USAging Eldercare

Many of these resources are available 24/7 and offer support in multiple languages. *If you're feeling overwhelmed, the Alzheimer's Association 24/7 Helpline at 800.272.3900 is available around the clock, 365 days a year, Alzheimer's Help & Support Alzheimer's Association and can provide immediate support and local resource referrals.*

About the Author

Dr. Patricia A. Farrell is a licensed psychologist, published author of multiple self-help books and videos, former WebMD psychologist expert/consultant, medical consultant for Social Security Disability Determinations, Alzheimer's psychiatric researcher at Mt. Sinai Medical Center (NYC), an educator who has taught at the college, graduate, and postgraduate levels, and a top health writer for *Medium.com* publications.

Her influence extends to the pharmaceutical and marketing industries, where she serves as a consultant and has appeared on major TV news programs in the US and abroad. In addition, Dr. Farrell provides continuing education modules for mental healthcare professionals and has contributed to USMLE medical school prep courses. She shares her knowledge through her YouTube channel and her daily contributions to **Bluesky** (@carpenter22,bsky.social). Dr. Farrell's achievements are recognized in *Who's Who in the World, Who's Who in America,* and *Who's Who in American Women*.

A member of the American Psychological Association and the SAG-AFTRA union, Dr. Farrell is a former board member of the NJ Board of Psychological Examiners, a former psychiatry preceptor at

UMDNJ, and a former board of directors member of Bergen Pines Hospital (now Bergen Regional Hospital).

Books by Patricia A. Farrell, Ph.D.

How to Be Your Own Therapist

It's Not All in Your Head: Anxiety, Depression, Mood Swings and Multiple Sclerosis

Unfiltered: Beneath the noise of our thoughts lies the true narrative of our minds

Unfiltered Again: A behind-the-scenes look at healthcare, medicine and mental health

A Social Security Disability Psychological Claims Handbook: A simple guide to understanding your SSD claim for psychological impairments and unraveling the maze of decision-making

A Social Security Disability Psychological Claims Guidebook for Children's Benefits

The Disability Accessible US Parks in All 50 States: A Comprehensive Guide

Birding in the US NOW!: A birding guide for individuals with disabilities

A Special Request

I f this book has touched your heart, sparked your curiosity, or simply entertained you along the way, I'd be incredibly grateful if you could take a moment to share your thoughts with a review on Amazon or wherever you discovered this book. Your words not only help other readers find books they'll love, but they also mean the world to authors like me who pour their hearts into every page. Thank you for being part of this journey, and for helping stories find their way to the readers who need them most.